Cook Like a Pro

Air Fryer Toaster Oven

50 Recipes to Make Very Delicious

Dishes with Your Air Fryer and

Leave Everyone Impressed with

Your Cooking Skills

By

Linda Lavis

Table of Contents

Chapter 3: Snacks, Appetizers, and Sides 36

Introduction

Oil frying is a method of cooking in a fatty medium such as oil or animal fats that gives foods a crispy texture on the surface. An air fryer, however, achieves a texture and flavor similar to that of fried foods but with just a tablespoon of oil. This is why we get "fried" food but much healthier.

To get the best out of that air fryer you have at home, keep in mind the following tips:

- Stop frying only potatoes: Preparing french fries and saving excessive amounts of oil made this appliance so popular. However, everything can be fried: from sweet potatoes to kale chips. Be creative and take advantage of your fryer with other ingredients to accompany your dishes.

- Avoid moisture as much as possible: To get that crunchy texture, drain the food well before placing it in the fryer for best results.

- Fry in small quantities, like the food, will look better if you allow the air to circulate better and the heat to reach the entire surface of the food. You will have a better texture in your preparations. Do not exceed the quantities recommended by the manufacturer of your air fryer!

- To get that texture of fried food, you need to use oil. This is what will give the food a spectacular flavor, provide a crispy texture and promote the Maillard

reaction in our food.

So, what do you fancy frying with this appliance? With

this recipe booklet, you will have plenty of options to

get you started!

Chapter 1: Breakfast and

Brunch Recipes

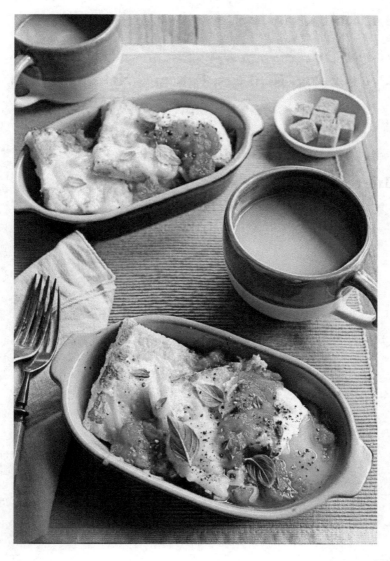

1. Simple Spaghetti Squash

(Ready in about 1 hour 35 minutes | **Serving:** 6 |

Difficulty: Hard)

Per serving: **Kcal** 223, **Fat**: 16 g, **Net Carbs**: 21 g,

Protein: 1 g

Ingredients:

- 2 lbs. seeded spaghetti squash, halved

- ½ cup butter, 10 equal chunks

- 4 tablespoons brown sugar, divided

- 2 tablespoons ground cinnamon, divided

Instructions:

1. Preheat the air fryer to 350°F. Place halves of spaghetti squash on the pan and add five butter pieces into each half. Add 2 tablespoons of sugar and 1 tablespoon of cinnamon on every half. Cook for around 1 hour. Take out of the fryer and scrape the insides using a fork, and cook for 10 more minutes.

2. Mushroom Quiche

(Ready in about 20 minutes | **Serving:** 4 | **Difficulty**:

Easy)

Per serving: Kcal 212, **Fat**: 4 g, **Net Carbs**: 7 g,

Protein: 7 g

Ingredients:

- 1 tablespoon flour

- 1 tablespoon butter, soft

- 9" pie dough

- 2 chopped button mushrooms

- 2 tablespoons chopped ham

- 3 eggs

- 1 small chopped yellow onion

- 1/3 cup heavy cream

- A pinch of ground nutmeg

- Salt and black pepper as per taste

- ½ teaspoon thyme, dried

- ¼ cup grated Swiss cheese

Instructions:

1. Add flour to the surface where you are working and roll dough. Add to the pan and mix the rest of the ingredients except Swiss cheese in a bowl. Pour over the dough and sprinkle on top Swiss cheese. Place pan in the fryer and cook for around 10 minutes at 400°F.

3. Corn Flakes Casserole

(Ready in about 18 minutes | **Serving**: 5 | **Difficulty**:

Easy)

Per serving: **Kcal** 300, **Fat**: 5 g, **Net Carbs**: 16 g,

Protein: 4 g

Ingredients:

- 1/3 cup milk

- 3 teaspoons sugar

- 2 whisked eggs

- ¼ teaspoon nutmeg, ground

- ¼ cup blueberries

- 4 tablespoons whipped cream cheese

- 1½ cups crumbled corn flakes

- 5 slices bread

Instructions:

1. Mix sugar, eggs, milk, and nutmeg in a bowl. Mix blueberries and cream cheese in another bowl. Add corn flakes to another bowl. Pour blueberry mixture on every slice of bread and dip in a mixture of eggs. Dredge in the corn flakes at the end and place them in the basket of the fryer. Heat to 400°F and cook for around 8 minutes.

4. Biscuits Casserole

(Ready in about 25 minutes | **Serving:** 8 | **Difficulty**:

Easy)

Per serving: Kcal 321, **Fat:** 4 g, **Net Carbs**: 12 g,

Protein: 5 g

Ingredients:

- 12 oz. biscuits, quartered

- 3 tablespoons flour

- ½ lb. sausage, chopped

- A pinch of black pepper and salt

- 2½ cup milk

- Cooking spray

Instructions:

1. Use cooking spray on the basket of air fryer and preheat to 350°F. Add biscuits at the base and mix the sausage. Add the rest of the ingredients and cook for around 15 minutes.

5. Best Pudding & Vanilla Sauce

(Ready in about 1 hour 25 minutes | **Serving:** 8 | **Difficulty**: Hard)

Per serving: Kcal 546, **Fat**: 17 g, **Net Carbs**: 92 g, **Protein**: 11 g

Ingredients:

- 4 beaten eggs

- 1 ½ cups refined sugar

- ¼ cup + 2 tablespoons melted butter

- 3 cups full-fat milk

- 10 slices farmhouse-style hearty bread, cubed and cooked

- 1 cup raisins

- ½ cup + 2 tablespoons light brown sugar

- 1 tablespoon white flour

- ½ teaspoon ground cinnamon, more if needed

- 1 ¼ cups full-fat milk

- A pinch of salt

- 1 tablespoon vanilla extract

Instructions:

1. Preheat the air fryer to 375°F. Oil a pan gently. Add half teaspoon cinnamon, a quarter cup of butter, 3 cups of milk, 3 eggs, 2 tablespoons of brown sugar, and white sugar, and add bread

cubes in a bowl and mix thoroughly, so everything is well incorporated. Pour this mixture on the pan and cook for around 55 minutes.

2. To create a sauce, mix the rest of the ingredients in a pan and warm on a moderate flame. Pour sauce on the bread pudding and enjoy.

Chapter 2: Fish and

Seafood Recipes

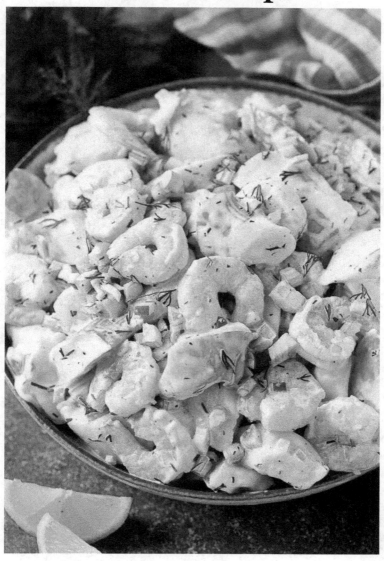

6. Salmon & Chives Vinaigrette

(Ready in about 22 minutes | **Serving:** 4 | **Difficulty:**

Easy)

Per serving: **Kcal:** 270, **Fat:** 3 g, **Net Carbs**: 25 g,

Protein: 10 g

Ingredients:

- 2 tablespoons dill, chopped

- 4 boneless salmon fillets

- 2 tablespoon chopped chives

- 1/3 cup maple syrup

- 1 tablespoon olive oil

- 3 tablespoons balsamic vinegar

- Salt

- Black pepper

Instructions:

1. Season fish using pepper and salt and rub oil over fish. Place in the fryer and broil for around 8 minutes at 350°F. Place a pot on flame and add the rest of the ingredients and cook for around 3 minutes. Serve on the side with fish and enjoy.

7. Swordfish & Mango Salsa

(Ready in about 16 minutes | **Serving:** 2 | **Difficulty**:

Easy)

Per serving: **Kcal**: 200, **Fat**: 7 g, **Net Carbs**: 14 g,

Protein: 14 g

Ingredients:

- 2 medium swordfish steaks

- Salt

- Black pepper

- 2 teaspoons avocado oil

- 1 tablespoon cilantro, chopped

- 1 chopped mango

- 1 chopped avocado, peeled and pitted

- A pinch of cumin

- A pinch of onion powder

- A pinch of garlic powder

- 1 sliced and peeled orange

- ½ tablespoon balsamic vinegar

Instructions:

1. Add seasonings to fish and rub with half the quantity of oil in a bowl. Place in pan and put it inside the fryer. Broil for around 6 minutes at 360°F. In the meantime, mix the rest of the ingredients in a bowl with the remaining oil to form salsa. Top fish with salsa and enjoy.

8. Roasted Cod & Prosciutto

(Ready in about 20 minutes | **Serving:** 4 | **Difficulty**:

Easy)

Per serving: Kcal: 200, **Fat:** 4 g, **Net Carbs**: 12 g,

Protein: 6 g

Ingredients:

- 1 tablespoon chopped parsley

- 4 medium cod filets

- ¼ cup melted butter

- 2 minced garlic cloves

- 2 tablespoon lemon juice

- 3 tablespoon prosciutto, chopped

- 1 teaspoon Dijon mustard

- 1 chopped shallot

- Salt

- Black pepper

Instructions:

1. Add all the ingredients except fish, pepper, and salt in a bowl and toss to combine evenly. Season fish using pepper and salt and spread bowl mixture over. Transfer to a pan and broil in the fryer for around 10 minutes at 390°F.

9. Marinated Salmon

(Ready in about 1 hour 20 minutes | **Serving:** 6 |

Difficulty: Hard)

Per serving: Kcal: 300, **Fat:** 8 g, **Net Carbs**: 19 g,

Protein: 27 g

Ingredients:

- 1 salmon, whole

- 1 tablespoon minced garlic

- 2 lemons juice

- 1 sliced lemon

- Salt

- Black pepper

Instructions:

1. Mix pepper, salt, lemon juice, and fish in a bowl and place in the fridge for an hour. Stuff salmon with lemon slices and garlic and place in the basket of the fryer. Broil for around 25 minutes at 320°F.

10. Salmon & Orange Marmalade

(Ready in about 25 minutes | **Serving:** 4 | **Difficulty**:

Easy)

Per serving: **Kcal**: 240, **Fat**: 9 g, **Net Carbs**: 14 g,

Protein: 10 g

Ingredients:

- 1 lb. wild salmon, skinless, cubed, and boneless

- 2 sliced lemons

- ¼ cup balsamic vinegar

- ¼ cup orange juice

- 1/3 cup orange marmalade

- A pinch of black pepper and salt

Instructions:

1. Warm vinegar in a pot and add orange juice and marmalade. Stir and simmer for around 1 minute. Thread lemon slices and salmon cubes on skewers and season using black pepper and salt. Brush them with half quantity of marmalade mix and place in the basket of the fryer. Broil for around 3 minutes at 360°F at one side. Brush remaining vinegar mix on skewers and enjoy.

Chapter 3: Snacks,

Appetizers, and Sides

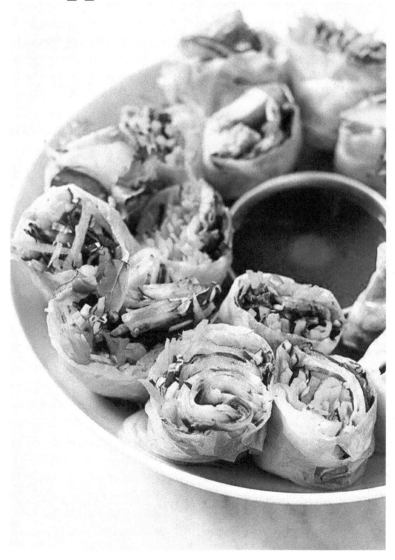

11. Potato Skins Strips

(Ready in about 20 minutes | **Serving:** 2 | **Difficulty:**

Easy)

Per serving: **Kcal:** 124, **Fat:** 4.8 g, **Net Carbs:** 16.6

g, **Protein:** 2.3 g

Ingredients:

- 2 baked medium russet potatoes

- Melted butter

- Seasoned salt

- Shredded cheese

Instructions:

1. Preheat the fryer to 450°F. Slice potatoes

   lengthwise in half and make a shell by scooping

potato flesh out. Brush shells with butter and place in a pan. Season and cook for around 10 minutes. Enjoy with dips of your choice.

12. Cooker Oven Potato Skins

(Ready in about 75 minutes | **Serving**: 4 | **Difficulty**: Hard)

Per serving: **Kcal:** 196, **Fat**: 5.8 g, **Net Carbs**: 31.8 g, **Protein**: 5.6 g

Ingredients:

- 4 small scrubbed russet potatoes, dried

- 4 teaspoons grapeseed oil

- 1/8 teaspoon smoked paprika

- Sea salt

- Black pepper

- ½ cup cheese, shredded

- 3 tablespoons plain non-fat Greek yogurt

- 1 finely sliced green onion

Instructions:

1. Preheat the fryer to 400°F. Stab potato with the fork on each side and rub 1 teaspoon oil. Place on a pan and cook for around 45 minutes. Slice potatoes lengthwise in half and scoop flesh out, making the shell of 1/4 inch. Combine paprika and the rest of the oil. Brush the skin of the potato with oil and season using pepper and salt. Place flesh and potato halves in the pan and

cook for 12 minutes. Fill the skins with cheese and top with onion and yogurt.

13. Bagel Chips

(Ready in about 25 minutes | **Serving**: 3 | **Difficulty**: Easy)

Per serving: **Kcal:** 137, **Fat**: 3 g, **Net Carbs**: 19.7 g, **Protein**: 4 g

Ingredients:

- 1 bagel, unsliced

- 1 tablespoon olive oil

- Sea salt

Instructions:

1. Preheat the fryer to 350°F. Slice the bagel into pieces 1/4 inch thick. Add slices to a bowl and add oil and salt. Mix thoroughly and arrange pieces on the pan. Cook for around 10 minutes. Flip and cook for 8 more minutes.

14. Potato Wedges

(Ready in about 40 minutes | **Serving**: 3 | **Difficulty**: Moderate)

Per serving: **Kcal**: 256, **Fat**: 5 g, **Net Carbs**: 46 g, **Protein**: 5 g

Ingredients:

- 3 teaspoon oil

- 12 oz. scrubbed russet potatoes, wedged

- 1 tablespoon seasoning everything bagel

Instructions:

1. Preheat the fryer to 400°F. Add 1 teaspoon oil to the pan. Toss potatoes with the rest of the oil in a bowl and add seasoning. Place wedges in one layer and cook for around 15 minutes. Tip all wedges onto their sides with a fork and cook for 15 more minutes.

15. Macaroni & Cheese

(Ready in about 40 minutes | **Serving**: 3 | **Difficulty**: Easy)

Per serving: **Kcal:** 341, **Fat**: 7 g, **Net Carbs**: 18 g, **Protein**: 4 g

Ingredients:

- 1½ cups any macaroni

- Cooking spray

- ½ cup heavy cream

- 1 cup chicken stock

- ¾ cup shredded cheddar cheese

- ½ cup shredded mozzarella cheese

- ¼ cup shredded parmesan

- Salt

- Black pepper

Instructions:

1. Apply cooking spray to the pan and add all the ingredients. Place pan in the basket of air fryer and cook for around 30 minutes. Divide among plates and eat.

16. Kale Chips

(Ready in about 20 minutes | **Serving**: 2 | **Difficulty**: Easy)

Per serving: **Kcal:** 52, **Fat**: 2.9 g, **Net Carbs**: 5.9 g, **Protein**: 2.9 g

Ingredients:

- 1 large kale leaf

- Cooking sprays

- sea salt

Additional Options for Seasoning:

- Lemon peel freshly, grated

- Seasoned salt

- Any Seasoning Mix

Instructions:

1. Preheat the fryer to 300°F. Wash leaves of kale and dry. Remove large ribs and thick stems. Arrange on a pan and spray oil. Sprinkle with lemon zest and sea salt. Cook for around 6 minutes and rotate pieces to cook for 5 more minutes.

17. Pita Chips

(Ready in about 14 minutes | **Serving**: 2 | **Difficulty**:

Easy)

Per serving: **Kcal**: 180, **Fat**: 2.8 g, **Net Carbs**: 35.3

g, **Protein**: 6.3 g

Ingredients:

- 2 whole-wheat mini pitas

- 1 teaspoon olive oil

- Sea salt

Instructions:

1. Preheat the fryer to 375°F. Brush oil on pitas

   and sprinkle seasoning. Slice pitas into four

wedges. Place on a pan and cook for around 9 minutes. They will turn crispy and golden.

18. Sweet Potato Nachos

(Ready in about 35 minutes | **Serving**: 2 | **Difficulty**: Easy)

Per serving: **Kcal**: 299, **Fat**: 14.5 g, **Net Carbs**: 34 g, **Protein**: 10.2 g

Ingredients:

- 6 oz. sweet potato, ½" thick slices

- 2 teaspoon olive oil

- Salt and pepper

- 1 thinly sliced jalapeño

- ¼ cup refried beans vegetarian

- 1 tablespoon enchilada sauce

- ¼ cup drained canned corn

- ½ cup cheese shredded

Optional Toppings:

- Chopped cilantro

- Lime wedges

- Green onions

- Chopped tomatoes

- Guacamole

- Salsa

Instructions:

1. Preheat the fryer to 425°F. Place slices of potato in an even layer on the pan. Sprinkle with pepper and salt and brush using oil. Cook for around 10 minutes. Mix enchilada sauce and beans in a bowl. Add mixture to pan and top with jalapeno slices, cheese, and corn. Cook for around 5 more minutes.

19. Balsamic Cranberries

(Ready in about 28 minutes | **Serving**: 3 | **Difficulty**:

Easy)

Per serving: **Kcal**: 36, **Fat**: 0.7 g, **Net Carbs**: 7.5 g,

Protein: 0.1 g

Ingredients:

- 8 oz. fresh cranberries

- 3 tablespoon maple syrup, real

- 2 tablespoon balsamic vinegar

- ½ teaspoon orange peel, grated

- 1 tablespoon orange juice

- 1 ½ teaspoon EVOO

- 1/8 teaspoon sea salt

- A pinch of black pepper

Instructions:

1. Preheat the fryer to 425°F. Add cranberries to a pan and place them aside. Mix the rest of the ingredients in a bowl and pour the mixture over cranberries. Stir thoroughly and cover the pan. Cook for around 15 minutes and stir after every 5 minutes.

20. Strawberry Salsa with Cinnamon Chips

(Ready in about 17 minutes | **Serving**: 2 | **Difficulty**: Easy)

Per serving: Kcal: 120, **Fat:** 2.1 g, **Net Carbs:** 25.3

g, **Protein:** 2.2 g

Ingredients:

Baked Cinnamon Tortilla Chips:

- 2 (8") corn tortillas

- ½ teaspoon coconut oil, melted

- ¼ teaspoon cinnamon

- ¼ teaspoon coconut sugar

- 1/8 teaspoon sea salt

Strawberry Salsa:

- ½ cup strawberries, finely chopped

- ½ teaspoon honey

- ¼ teaspoon lime peel, freshly grated

- 1 tablespoon lime juice

- 1/3 cup mango, finely chopped

- 1/3 cup jicama, finely chopped

Instructions:

1. Preheat the fryer to 425°F. Combine salt, cinnamon, and coconut sugar in a bowl. Stack tortillas on one another and dice into 8 triangles. Coat each piece with oil. Sprinkle bowl mixture on it and cook for around 7 minutes. Mix 2 tablespoons of strawberries, lime peel, honey, and lime juice in a bowl. Make a sauce and add mango, jicama, and the rest of the strawberries. Serve salsa with tortilla chips.

Chapter 4: Beef Recipes

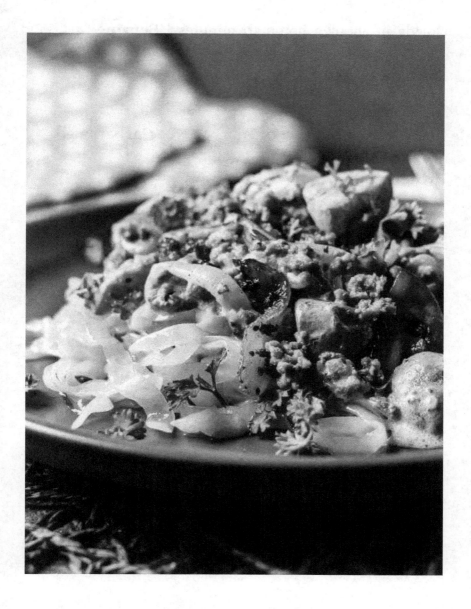

21. Medallions

(Ready in about 2 hours 10 minutes | **Serving**: 4 |

Difficulty: Hard)

Per serving: Kcal: 230, **Fat**: 4 g, **Net Carbs**: 13 g,

Protein: 14 g

Ingredients:

- 2 teaspoons chili powder

- 1 cup crushed tomatoes

- 4 beef medallions

- 2 teaspoons onion powder

- 2 tablespoons soy sauce

- Black pepper and salt

- 1 tablespoon hot pepper

- 2 tablespoons lime juice

Instructions:

1. Add all the ingredients except beef in a bowl and mix thoroughly. Arrange beef in a pan and pour sauce. Place aside for around 10 minutes. Discard marinade of tomatoes and broil for around 10 minutes at 360°F.

22. Jerky Beef

(Ready in about 3 hours 30 minutes | **Serving:** 6 |

Difficulty: Hard)

Per serving: **Kcal:** 300, **Fat:** 12 g, **Net Carbs:** 3 g,

Protein: 8 g

Ingredients:

- 2 cups soy sauce

- ½ cup Worcestershire sauce

- 2 tablespoons black peppercorns

- 2 tablespoons black pepper

- 2 lbs. sliced beef round

Instructions:

1. Mix everything in a bowl and place in the fridge for around 6 hours. Take out and place in a basket and broil for 1 and a half hours at 370°F. Move mixture to a bowl and serve chilled.

23. Beef Rolls

(Ready in about 24 minutes | **Serving:** 4 | **Difficulty**: Easy)

Per serving: **Kcal**: 230, **Fat**: 1 g, **Net Carbs**: 12 g, **Protein**: 10 g

Ingredients:

- 2 lbs. flattened opened beef steak, with tenderizer

- Salt

- Black pepper

- 1 cup spinach

- 3 oz. chopped bell pepper, roasted

- 6 provolone cheese slices

- 3 tablespoons pesto

Instructions:

1. Spread cheese and pesto over steak and add pepper, spinach, salt, and bell pepper. Roll the steak and insert toothpicks. Season with more pepper and salt. Place the roll in the basket and broil for around 14 minutes at 400°F. Flip midway.

Chapter 5: Bakery and

Desserts

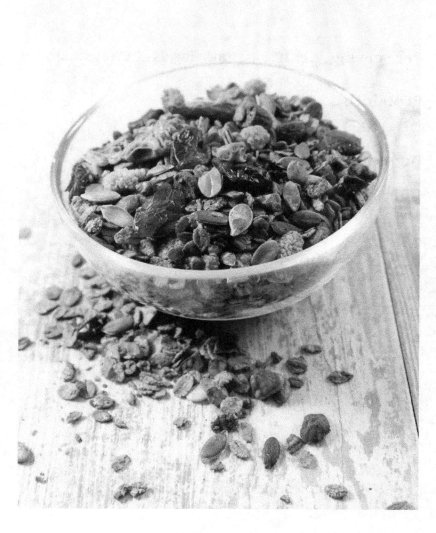

24. Crunchy Granola

(Ready in about 35 minutes | **Serving:** 4 | **Difficulty**:

Easy)

Per serving: **Kcal:** 290, **Fat**: 18 g, **Net Carbs**: 29 g,

Protein: 6 g

Ingredients:

- 1½ cup rolled oats

- ¾ cup nuts, raw

- ½ cup shredded unsweetened coconut

- ¼ cup sunflower seeds, hulled

- ¼ cup pumpkin seeds, hulled

- ¼ cup melted coconut oil

- ¼ cup maple syrup, pure

- ½ teaspoon kosher salt

- ¼ teaspoon ground cinnamon

- A pinch of powdered nutmeg

- ½ cup fruit dried

Instructions:

1. Prepare the pan with parchment paper. Mix all the ingredients except dried fruits. Pour this in the pan and bake for 20 minutes at 300°F. Add the dried fruits and cool.

25. "Fried" Apples

(Ready in about 15 minutes | **Serving:** 2 | **Difficulty**:

Easy)

Per serving: **Kcal:** 126, **Fat:** 4 g, **Net Carbs**: 22 g,

Protein: 1 g

Ingredients:

- ½ sliced apple

- 1 tablespoon melted unsalted butter

- 1/3 cup graham cracker crumbs

Instructions:

1. Prepare the pan. Spread apples in the pan and

   add butter and graham cracker crumbs to them.

Bake for 10 minutes at 400°F until brown.

Serve.

26. Peanut Butter Brownies

(Ready in about 25 minutes | **Serving:** 16 | **Difficulty**: Easy)

Per serving: Kcal: 317, **Fat:** 21 g, **Net Carbs**: 32 g, **Protein**: 5 g

Ingredients

- Non-stick spray

- ¾ cup cubed unsalted butter

- 4 oz. chopped unsweetened chocolate

- 4 oz. chopped bittersweet chocolate

- 2 tablespoons cocoa powder

- 2 teaspoons espresso powder

- 3 eggs

- 1½ cups granulated sugar

- 2 teaspoons vanilla extract, pure

- ½ cup all-purpose unbleached flour

- ¾ teaspoon kosher salt

- ½ cup peanut butter

- ¼ cup sifted confectioners' sugar

- 2 tablespoons melted unsalted butter, cooled

- A pinch of kosher salt

Instructions:

1. Prepare the pan with parchment paper and oil. Melt butter, chocolate, cocoa powder, and espresso powder over boiling water. Mix the rest of the ingredients in a bowl and add the chocolate mixture to that. For peanut butter, mix peanut butter, confectioners' sugar, and melted butter. Now bake the mixture for 25 minutes at 350°F. Cool and serve.

27. Egg Bagel

(Ready in about 35 minutes | **Serving:** 2 | **Difficulty**:

Easy)

Per serving: Kcal: 52, **Fat**: 25 g, **Net Carbs**: 56 g,

Protein: 22 g

Ingredients:

- 2 split bagels

- 2 teaspoons butter, softened

- 3 sprays cooking oil, non-stick

- 2 eggs

- 2 teaspoons sriracha sauce

- 1 oz. cheese, thinly sliced divided

- 1 small pitted avocado, mashed

- 1/3 cup sliced grape tomatoes

- ½ cup roughly chopped arugula

- Salt

- Pepper

Instructions:

1. Cut open the bagels to separate the interior bread from the crust. Now spread the interior with butter to bake them. Prepare the bagel halves with sauce and cheese. Preheat the fryer at 350°F and oil it. Break the eggs in the fryer cavity and tear the yolk and sprinkle salt and pepper. Bake these eggs for 8 to 11 minutes. Mix mashed avocado, sliced tomatoes, arugula, salt,

and pepper. Now put the egg, avocado mixture in between the bagel halves and serve.

28. Sweet Popcorn

(Ready in about 15 minutes | **Serving:** 4 | **Difficulty**: Easy)

Per serving: **Kcal:** 70, **Fat:** 0.2 g, **Net Carbs**: 1 g, **Protein**: 1 g

Ingredients:

- 2 tablespoons corn kernels

- 2 ½ tablespoons butter

- 2 oz. brown sugar

Instructions:

1. Bake the corns at 400°F in a fryer. Melt sugar in butter in a pan. Pour corns in this melted butter. Cool and serve.

29. Light Cookies

(Ready in about 15 minutes | **Serving:** 1 | **Difficulty:** Easy)

Per serving: Kcal: 528, **Fat:** 29 g, **Net Carbs:** 62 g, **Protein:** 6 g

Ingredients:

- 2 tablespoons butter, softened

- 2 tablespoons dark brown firmly packed sugar

- 1 tablespoon granulated sugar

- A pinch of kosher salt

- ¼ teaspoon vanilla extract, pure

- 1 yolk

- ¼ teaspoon baking soda

- ¼ cup white flour

- 3 tablespoons semi-sweet chocolate chips

Instructions:

1. Preheat the fryer at 350°F and oil the pan. Mix all the ingredients in a bowl. Spread the cookies on the pan and sprinkle chocolate chips on them and bake for 10 minutes until golden brown. Cool and serve.

30. Bourbon Brownies

(Ready in about 50 minutes | **Serving:** 4 | **Difficulty:**

Moderate)

Per serving: **Kcal:** 342, **Fat:** 22 g, **Net Carbs:** 37 g,

Protein: 4 g

Ingredients:

- 6 tablespoons unsalted butter

- 6 oz. semi-sweet chocolate chips

- ¼ cup cocoa powder, unsweetened

- ¾ cup white flour

- ¼ teaspoon baking powder

- ¼ teaspoon salt

- 1 cup light brown packed sugar

- 2 eggs

- ¼ cup bourbon

- 2 teaspoons vanilla extract, pure

- ½ cup unsalted roasted pecans, coarsely chopped

Instructions:

1. Preheat the fryer to 350°F. Coat pan with some butter. Mix butter, cocoa, and chocolate in a bowl. Place over pan having simmering water. Stir until chocolate and butter melts. Mix baking powder, flour, and salt in another bowl. Add sugar, bourbon, eggs, and vanilla in an electric mixer and beat on moderate speed for around 4 minutes. Add the mixture of chocolate and combine. Add pecans and pour the mixture on the pan. Bake for around 35 minutes.

Chapter 6: Pork and Lamb

Recipes

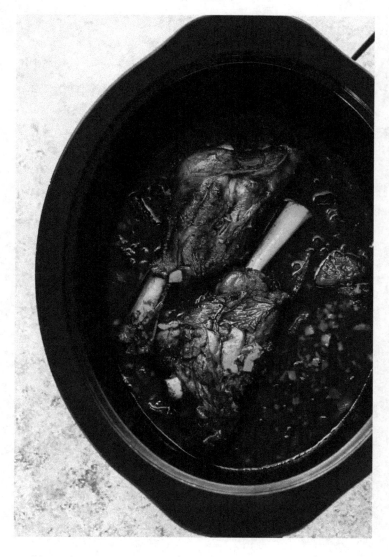

31. Creamy Pork

(Ready in about 32 minutes | **Serving:** 6 | **Difficulty**: Easy)

Per serving: **Kcal:** 300, **Fat:** 10 g, **Net Carbs**: 26 g, **Protein**: 34 g

Ingredients:

- 2 lbs. boneless pork meat cubed

- 2 chopped yellow onions

- 1 tablespoon olive oil

- 1 minced garlic clove

- 3 cups chicken stock

- 2 tablespoons sweet paprika

- Black pepper and salt

- 2 tablespoons white flour

- 1 1/2 cups sour cream

- 2 tablespoons chopped dill

Instructions:

1. Mix pork with pepper, salt, and oil in a pan. Place in fryer and toast for around 7 minutes at 360°F. Add the rest of the ingredients to the pan and toast for around 15 minutes at 370°F.

32. Pork with Onions

(Ready in about 1 day 25 minutes | **Serving:** 6 |

Difficulty: Hard)

Per serving: **Kcal:** 384, **Fat**: 4 g, **Net Carbs**: 17 g,

Protein: 25 g

Ingredients:

- 2 pork chops

- 1/4 cup olive oil

- 2 sliced yellow onions

- 2 minced garlic cloves

- 2 teaspoons mustard

- 1 teaspoon sweet paprika

- Black pepper and salt

- 1/2 teaspoon dried oregano

- 1/2 teaspoon dried thyme

- A pinch of pepper

Instructions:

1. Add all the ingredients except meat and onions in a bowl. Whisk to make a mixture. Add meat and onions and toss so it is coated thoroughly. Cover and place in the fridge for around 1 day. Transfer mixture to a pan and place in fryer. Toast for around 25 minutes at 360°F.

33. Pork Shoulder

(Ready in about 1 hour 50 minutes | **Serving:** 6 |

Difficulty: Hard)

Per serving: **Kcal:** 221, **Fat**: 4 g, **Net Carbs**: 7 g,

Protein: 10 g

Ingredients:

- 3 tablespoons minced garlic

- 3 tablespoons olive oil

- 4 lbs. pork shoulder

- Black pepper and salt

Instructions:

1. Add all the ingredients to a bowl and mix. Add pork and coat with mixture. Place in a pan and toast for around 10 minutes at 390°F. Reduce temperature to 300°F and toast for around an hour.

34. Sausage with Mushrooms

(Ready in about 50 minutes | **Serving:** 6 | **Difficulty**:

Moderate)

Per serving: **Kcal:** 130, **Fat**: 12 g, **Net Carbs**: 13 g,

Protein: 18 g

Ingredients:

- 3 chopped red bell peppers

- 2 lbs. sliced pork sausage

- Black pepper and salt

- 2 lbs. sliced Portobello mushrooms

- 2 chopped sweet onions

- 1 tablespoon brown sugar

- 1 teaspoon olive oil

Instructions:

1. Add sausages with the rest of the ingredients in a pan. Toss to combine the ingredients and coat sausages thoroughly. Bake for around 40 minutes at 300°F.

Chapter 7: Poultry Recipes

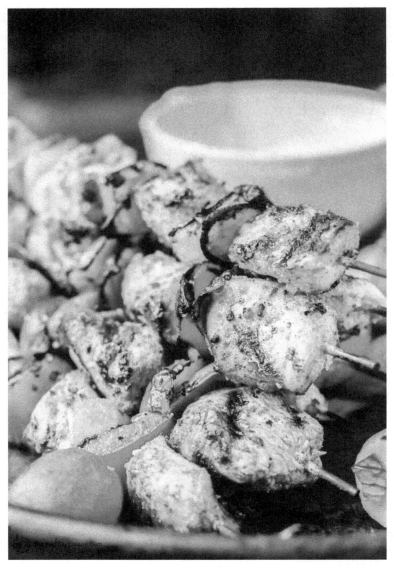

35. Chicken Kabobs

(Ready in about 30 minutes | **Serving:** 2 | **Difficulty:**

Easy)

Per serving: **Kcal:** 261, **Fat:** 7 g, **Net Carbs**: 12 g,

Protein: 6 g

Ingredients:

- 3 squared cut orange bell pepper

- ¼ cup honey

- 1/3 cup soy sauce

- Salt

- Black pepper

- 6 halved mushrooms

- 2 boneless, skinless chicken breasts, roughly cubed

Instructions:

1. Add chicken, pepper, honey, soya sauce, salt in a bowl and mix it. Strand chicken, bell peppers and mushrooms on skewers, put them in fryer and toast at 338°F for around 20 minutes.

36. Delicious Wings

(Ready in about 55 minutes | **Serving:** 4 | **Difficulty:**

Moderate)

Per serving: Kcal: 271, **Fat:** 6 g, **Net Carbs**: 18 g,

Protein: 18 g

Ingredients:

- 3 lbs. chicken wings

- ½ cup butter

- 1 tablespoon Old Bay® seasoning

- ¾ cup potato starch

- 1 teaspoon lemon juice

- Lemon wedges

Instructions:

1. Mix starch, Old Bay® seasoning and chicken wings and mix well. Put chicken wings in the fryer's basket and toast at 360°F for around 35 minutes. Increase temperature to 400°F, cook further for 10 minutes. Add butter to a pan and melt. Add butter and lemon over the chicken.

37. Hot Dogs

(Ready in about 17 minutes | **Serving:** 2 | **Difficulty**: Easy)

Per serving: Kcal: 211, **Fat:** 3 g, **Net Carbs**: 12 g, **Protein**: 4 g

Ingredients:

- 2 hot dog buns

- 2 hot dogs

- 1 tablespoon Dijon mustard

- 2 tablespoon grated cheddar cheese

Instructions:

1. Place hot dogs in the preheated fryer and toast
    them at 390°F for around 5 minutes. Put hot
    dogs in hot dog buns, put mustard and cheese
    toast in the fryer for further two minutes at
    390°F.

38. Tasty Ham with Greens

(Ready in about 26 minutes | **Serving:** 8 | **Difficulty:**

Easy)

Per serving: **Kcal:** 322, **Fat:** 6 g, **Net Carbs**: 12 g,

Protein: 5 g

Ingredients:

- 2 tablespoons olive oil

- 4 cups chopped ham

- 2 tablespoons flour

- 3 cups chicken stock

- 5 oz. chopped onion

- 16 oz. chopped collard greens

- 14 oz. canned drained black peas

- 1/2 teaspoon crushed red pepper

Instructions:

1. Warm oil in a pan and add flour, ham, and stock. Mix and add the rest of the ingredients and place them in a fryer. Toast for around 16 minutes at 390°F.

39. Japanese Mix

(Ready in about 18 minutes | **Serving:** 2 | **Difficulty**:

Easy)

Per serving: **Kcal:** 300, **Fat:** 7 g, **Net Carbs**: 17 g,

Protein: 10 g

Ingredients:

- 2 boneless and skinless chicken thighs

- 2 chopped ginger slices

- 3 minced garlic cloves

- ¼ cup soy sauce

- ¼ cup mirin

- ½ teaspoon sesame oil

- 1/8 cup water

- 2 tablespoons sugar

- 1 tablespoon cornstarch in 2 tablespoon water

Instructions:

1. Take chicken thighs, ginger, garlic, soy sauce, mirin, oil, water, sugar, and cornstarch and mix well. Put it in the preheated fryer and cook at 360°F for around 8 minutes.

40. Sweet and Sour Sausage

(Ready in about 20 minutes | **Serving:** 4 | **Difficulty**:

Easy)

Per serving: **Kcal:** 162, **Fat:** 6 g, **Net Carbs:** 12 g,

Protein: 6 g

Ingredients:

- 1 lb. sausages, sliced

- 1 striped cut red bell pepper

- ½ cup chopped yellow onion

- 3 tablespoons brown sugar

- 1/3 cup ketchup

- 2 tablespoons mustard

- 2 tablespoons cider vinegar

- ½ cup chicken stock

Instructions:

1. In a bowl, mix sugar with ketchup, mustard, stock, and vinegar and whisk well. In your air fryer's pan, mix sausage slices with bell pepper, onion, and sweet and sour mix, toss and cook at 350°F for 10 minutes. Divide into bowls and serve for lunch. Enjoy.

Chapter 8: Vegetable

Recipes

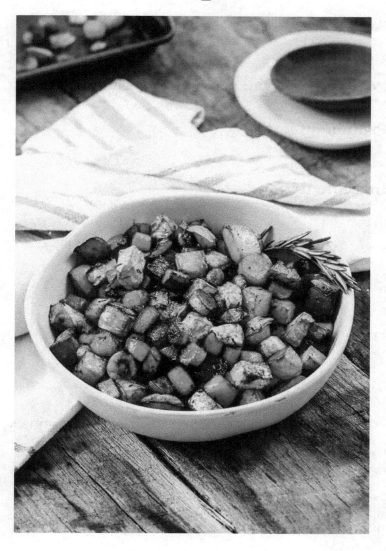

41. Eggplant with Tomato Toast

(Ready in about 45 minutes | **Serving:** 4 | **Difficulty**:

Easy)

Per serving: **Kcal:** 289, **Fat**: 11 g, **Net Carbs**: 40 g,

Protein: 10 g

Ingredients:

- 1 small diagonally cut eggplant, ¼" thick

- 8 thick Italian bread slices

- 1 pint grape or cherry tomatoes

- 1 medium finely minced garlic clove

- 3 tablespoons chopped fresh herbs (rosemary,

  marjoram, basil)

- ¼ cup olive oil

- Kosher salt

- Black pepper

- 8 oz. ricotta cheese

Instructions:

1. Preheat the fryer to 400°F. Mix 2 tablespoons of herbs, garlic, and oil in a bowl. Brush mixture over eggplant and season using pepper and salt. Repeat with slices of bread, add tomatoes with the rest of the oil, and mix. Season using pepper and salt. Place tomatoes in the basket and toast for around 15 minutes. Take tomatoes out on a plate. Place eggplant in basket and toast for around 13 minutes. Toast bread for around 5 minutes. Divide tomatoes and eggplant between

slices of bread and add ricotta on top sprinkle with fresh herbs.

42. Tofu with Shallots

(Ready in about 35 minutes | **Serving:** 4 | **Difficulty**: Easy)

Per serving: **Kcal:** 540, **Fat:** 23 g, **Net Carbs**: 57 g, **Protein**: 33 g

Ingredients:

- 1 lb. firm tofu block well-drained, patted dry (1" cubes)

- 4 shallots large halved lengthwise and sliced crosswise ½" thick slices

- 3 thinly sliced green onions

Sauce:

- 1 teaspoon finely minced garlic

- 1 teaspoon finely minced ginger

- ½ teaspoon black pepper

- ½ teaspoon sesame oil, toasted

- 1 tablespoon hoisin sauce

- 2 teaspoons soy sauce

- ½ teaspoon cornstarch

- ¼ cup water, chicken stock, or vegetable stock

- ¼ teaspoon cayenne pepper powder

Instructions:

1. Preheat fryer to 400°F. Add tofu cubes and shallots to the pan. Toast for around 15 minutes. Mix sauce ingredients in a bowl. Coat shallots and tofu with sauce and place in pan. Reduce temperature to 350°F and toast for around 5 minutes. Garnish with onions and enjoy.

43. Tofu

(Ready in about 45 minutes | **Serving:** 4 | **Difficulty**:

Easy)

Per serving: **Kcal:** 154, **Fat**: 13 g, **Net Carbs**: 1 g,

Protein: 11 g

Ingredients:

- 1 carrot, large

- 1 cup snow peas

- 1 lb. tofu, cut into ½" cubes

- ¼ cup separated sesame oil

- 2 tablespoons soy sauce

- 1 tablespoon sesame seeds

Instructions:

1. Peel lemon and dice into fine strips. Transfer to a bowl and add snow peas. Cut tofu into cubes of 1/2 inch. Add to carrot and peas. Add 3 tablespoons of oil and toss. Place in the basket of fryer and toast for around 30 minutes at 400°F. Mix rest of ingredients in a bowl and toss vegetable blend and tofu in it.

44. Jacket Potatoes

(Ready in about 25 minutes | **Serving:** 2 | **Difficulty**:

Easy)

Per serving: **Kcal:** 197, **Fat:** 7 g, **Net Carbs**: 13 g,

Protein: 8 g

Ingredients:

- 2 potatoes, medium-sized

- 1 teaspoon butter

- 3 tablespoons sour cream

- 1 teaspoon chives

- 2 tablespoons grated cheese

- Pepper and salt

Instructions:

1. Stab potatoes using a fork and place them in the basket of the fryer. Toast for around 15 minutes at 320°F. Mix the rest of the ingredients in the bowl in the meantime to make a filling for potatoes. Open potatoes and add butter and topping mixture and enjoy.

45. Arugula Salad

(Ready in about 20 minutes | **Serving:** 4 | **Difficulty**:

Easy)

Per serving: Kcal: 121, **Fat:** 2 g, **Net Carbs**: 11 g,

Protein: 4 g

Ingredients:

- 1 ½ lb. peeled beets, quartered

- A drizzle of olive oil

- 2 teaspoons grated orange zest

- 2 tablespoons cider vinegar

- 1/2 cup orange juice

- 2 tablespoons brown sugar

- 2 chopped scallions

- 2 teaspoons mustard

- 2 cups arugula

Instructions:

1. Add oil to beets and mix in orange juice. Place in pan and toast for around 10 minutes at 350°F. Add beets to bowl and add rest of ingredients except mustard, sugar, and vinegar. Toss to coat beets. Mix mustard, sugar, and vinegar in another bowl. Add to salad and toss.

46. Broccoli Salad

(Ready in about 18 minutes | **Serving:** 4 | **Difficulty:** Easy)

Per serving: **Kcal:** 121, **Fat:** 3 g, **Net Carbs**: 4 g, **Protein**: 4 g

Ingredients:

- 1 floret separated broccoli head

- 1 tablespoon peanut oil

- 6 minced garlic cloves

- 1 tablespoon rice vinegar

- Black pepper and salt

Instructions:

1. Mix broccoli with pepper, salt, and half the
   amount of oil in a bowl. Place in a pan and toast
   for around 8 minutes at 350°F. Transfer to a
   bowl and add the rest of the ingredients and
   toss.

47. Brussels Sprouts with Tomatoes

(Ready in about 15 minutes | **Serving:** 4 | **Difficulty:** Easy)

Per serving: Kcal: 121, **Fat:** 4 g, **Net Carbs:** 11 g, **Protein:** 4 g

Ingredients:

- 1 pound trimmed Brussels sprouts

- Black pepper and salt

- 6 halved cherry tomatoes

- 1/4 cup chopped green onions

- 1 tablespoon olive oil

Instructions:

1. Season sprouts with pepper and salt. Place in pan and toast for around 10 minutes at 350°F. Transfer to a bowl and add the rest of the ingredients. Toss to mix and enjoy.

48. Cheesy Sprouts

(Ready in about 18 minutes | **Serving:** 4 | **Difficulty**:

Easy)

Per serving: Kcal: 152, **Fat:** 6 g, **Net Carbs**: 8 g,

Protein: 12 g

Ingredients:

- 1 lb. washed Brussels sprouts

- 1 lemon juice

- Black pepper and salt

- 2 tablespoons butter

- 3 tablespoons grated parmesan

Instructions:

1. Toast sprouts for around 8 minutes at 350°F. Place in a bowl and warm a pan with butter over moderate flame. Add the rest of the ingredients except parmesan and whisk. Add sprouts and parmesan. Cook until cheese melts.

49. Spicy Cabbage

(Ready in about 18 minutes | **Serving:** 4 | **Difficulty**:

Easy)

Per serving: **Kcal:** 100, **Fat**: 4 g, **Net Carbs**: 11 g,

Protein: 7 g

Ingredients:

- 1 cabbage, diced into eight wedges

- 1 tablespoon sesame seed oil

- 1 grated carrot

- 1/4 cup apple vinegar

- 1/4 cups apple juice

- 1/2 teaspoon cayenne pepper

- 1 teaspoon crushed pepper flakes

Instructions:

1. Add oil to cabbage and mix the rest of the ingredients in a pan that can be placed in your fryer and toast for around 8 minutes at 350°F.

50. Sweet Carrots

(Ready in about 20 minutes | **Serving:** 4 | **Difficulty:**

Easy)

Per serving: **Kcal:** 100, **Fat:** 2 g, **Net Carbs:** 7 g,

Protein: 4 g

Ingredients:

- 2 cups baby carrots

- Black pepper and salt

- 1 tablespoon brown sugar

- 1/2 tablespoon melted butter

Instructions:

1. Add carrots to butter and mix the rest of the ingredients in a pan that can be placed in your fryer. Toast for around 10 minutes at 350°F.

Conclusion

Air fryers are increasingly used in food preparation due to their practicality, speed and what has made them popular: frying without oil, which allows a more nutritious and tasty food, with much fewer calories, cholesterol and fat.

In fact, meals prepared with an air fryer, whether fried, roasted, baked or toasted, bring us health benefits such as:

- Decreased fat consumption. The main reason people love the air fryer is that, compared to traditional frying, it significantly reduces total calorie intake by reducing the amount of oil used in the preparations.

- Decrease in calorie intake by about 70%, which will have an impact on weight loss or weight maintenance if a healthy diet is maintained.

- They make vegetables a more attractive food, which encourages their consumption.

And all this with the advantage of being able to prepare food faster than in a conventional oven and more easily. You don't need to be an expert in the kitchen to prepare great recipes for yourself and your loved ones.